Yoga for Beginners:
A Quick and Easy Guide to Start Your Yoga Journey

Emily McManson

Yoga for Beginners: A Quick and Easy Guide to Start Your Yoga Journey

Before beginning any new exercise program it is recommended that you seek medical advice from your personal physician.

ISBN: 1981260102
ISBN-13: 978-1981260102

CONTENTS

INTRODUCTION

All over the Western World people are trying yoga. Some come in hopes of dealing with the stress of their busy lives. Others try it in hopes of improved health and fitness. Regardless of the reason, yoga offers a wide array of benefits to all who practice. Yoga helps to strengthen the body while increasing flexibility and muscle tone. When paired with deep breathing, yoga can simultaneously relax and energize. Yoga can help release stress and detoxify your body. Its numerous health benefits make yoga an invaluable tool for you to use on the road to health and vitality.

Yoga gives us the opportunity to reconnect with our bodies, minds, and spirits. While we journey through this rat race of life, it is easy for these connections to fall by the wayside. By taking the time to develop a yoga practice, we give ourselves a gift that extends beyond any other exercise.

However, yoga can be a little intimidating at the beginning. In this book, we've put together all you need to know about yoga and how to get started on your yoga journey.

In this book, we will cover:

- What yoga is
- Different styles of yoga
- How you can use yoga to improve your health and fitness
- Yoga poses and sequences designed for beginners
- What you need to set up a home practice

WHAT IS YOGA?

Yoga originated in India, over 2,000 years ago by the sage, Patanjali. Within yoga, there are eight separate limbs, referred to as the 8 Limbs of Yoga. Of the 8 Limbs, the asana practice, or the physical poses, is just one limb.

Included in the other limbs are:
Ethical restraints (yamas)
Moral observances (niyamas)
Breathing techniques (pranayama)
Withdrawal of the senses (pratyahara)
Concentration (dharana)
Meditation (dhyana)
Full absorption of the practice (samadhi)

The word yoga means union. It refers to coming together of the body, mind, and spirit. Yogi's believe when all the 8 Limbs are practiced regularly, full enlightenment can be reached.

The Physical Practice

The poses in yoga help bring alignment to all parts of the body so that energy will flow more evenly. In yoga, it is believed that there are many energy channels in the body. By moving in the poses, the body will open, and energy will flow freely.

Regular practice of yoga poses helps to stretch and tone the body. Yoga poses purify through detoxifying movements. The poses can help the body by creating a more stable sense of strength and alignment. Additionally, yoga helps to calm and focus the mind. In yoga, there are many postures. Each type affects the body differently. When practiced in a sequence, the poses produce different effects.

Types of Yoga

There are many different styles of yoga. As a beginner, it is important to stick with one form of yoga as you familiarize yourself with the poses. As you progress in your practice, try different options out. To ease any confusion, we've given you an overview of some of the most popular styles of yoga.

Anusara - Founded by John Friend in 1997. Anusara offers rigorous, heart-themed classes. This style follows Friend's Universal Principles of Alignment.

Iyengar - Developed by BKS Iyengar, this style of yoga is the most alignment focused. This method uses many props, and a real Iyengar studio is full of bolsters, blocks, blankets, chairs, and even rope walls. The focus is on concentrating on the deep opening that comes from holding postures to find proper alignment.

Ashtanga - Ashtanga is a very rigorous and demanding style of yoga. Ashtanga consists of 6 different series. The various series follow the same poses in order every time. In Ashtanga, each pose is linked to one breath, making it a more fast-paced practice. Ashtanga is where Vinyasa originated.

Vinyasa - Vinyasa classes are full of free-flowing movement and give teachers an opportunity to hold innovative, unique classes. These classes can be fast-paced, offering students plenty of heart rate increasing movements. Vinyasa classes can be likened to dance, as students move smoothly throughout sequences.

Hatha - While Hatha is the third limb of the Yoga Sutras in which it refers to all asana practice, Hatha yoga labeled classes usually offer a gentle class comprised of beginner poses. This style of classes provide less of a workout but help you tap into the other highly desirable benefits of yoga.

Hot Yoga - Hot Yoga classes are held in a heated room. The sequences can be similar to Vinyasa styles or be a set sequence of poses. Many proponents of Hot Yoga believe the heated room loosens their muscles without much need for warm-up.

Restorative - Restorative classes offer an excellent way to achieve deep opening and relaxation. Usually supported by various props, students can expect to move slowly through poses without exerting too much energy. Restorative classes are a great way to recharge and let go of multiple stressors.

HOW TO START YOUR YOGA PRACTICE

Before starting, there are a few things to consider. If you are pregnant, have injuries, or high blood pressure, a practice should be modified or limited. It is important to check with a healthcare professional to see if you can practice or what you will want to exclude from your practice.

Yoga is unique to everyone – every BODY. Do what works for you. Take things slowly, doing what feels right. Modify each pose so that you can experience its benefits without pain or injury.

Once you are familiar with the poses and feel comfortable, increase intensity. When you are ready to take it to the next level, try moving faster, work harder versions of the poses, and experiment holding poses for an extended period (5 to 8 breaths).

Try committing to a regular practice if you want to see results. The more you practice, the better you'll get. Just be sure to listen to your body and take rest days. On days when you're feeling tired try a gentle practice.

Breathing

In addition to learning the poses, it is important to incorporate a specific type of breathing into the practice. Our breathing can change when we are overexerted. Throughout your practice, focus on keeping the breath slow and steady. Inhales should be deep(like when you take a deep breath before going underwater) and exhales full(like blowing up a balloon). When or if your breath becomes strained, concentrate on smoothing it out. This mindful breathing helps tremendously with creating a sense of calm and relaxation. Additionally, it can help in times of stress when you are not practicing yoga.

But I'm not flexible!

Yoga is for everyone. Everyone benefits from this practice. If flexibility is an issue, modify the poses. What works for one person may not work for another. Yoga is about respecting our bodies and listening to our individual needs.

Over time, you will see your body change. With a regular yoga practice you will be able to enjoy more mobility and begin to feel better.

Props

There are several different props you can use to assist your practice. Use yoga blocks to bring the floor closer to you or to prop up your seat. Blankets provide cushioning for the knees and are also great to use when propping up your seat. Straps help you reach your toes.

Starting a Home Practice

Starting a practice doesn't have to be complicated. The best place to start is to find a quiet space and roll out your yoga mat.

A complete practice will use different types of poses to help increase balance, strength, and flexibility. We have provided detailed descriptions of the yoga poses and have put together several sequences to practice. Be sure to include a long, restorative pose at the end. It is important because it allows effects of the practice to settle in and is very relaxing.

BEGINNER YOGA POSES

There are many, many yoga poses. Described below are several of the best poses for a beginner practice. Follow the instructions carefully and listen to your body as you move.

Standing Poses

<u>Mountain Pose</u>

- Stand at the front of mat with arms at sides. Even press into feet. Stand with big toes touching and heels slightly separated, or with feet hip distance.

- Straighten legs and lift kneecaps to activate leg muscles. Press evenly into feet.

- Tuck tailbone in slightly.

- Tilt pelvis, bringing it into a neutral position and draw belly in.

- Allow shoulder blades to move down back, away from ears. Keep arms straight, fingers extended, and triceps firm. Inner arms rotate slightly outward, so hands face forward.

Standing Forward Bend

- Stand in Mountain Pose, place hands on hips. Bend forward from hip joints. Draw belly in and lengthen the front torso as you fold forward.

- Knees bend slightly to accommodate tight hamstrings. Hands come to the floor just beyond the feet. Heels press firmly into the floor. Lift the tail bones toward the ceiling.

- Inhale and lift chest slightly. Exhale and relax into the pose. Allow head be relaxed.

- Remain here for 3 to 5 breaths.

- To return to a stand, bring hands to hips. Rise with a flat back.

<u>Upward Salute</u>

-   Stand in Mountain Pose. Arms turn outward.

-   Inhale and sweep arms toward the ceiling.

-   When arms reach overhead, press palms together and reach upward.

-   Shoulders move away from ears. Gaze up, tip the head back slightly.

-   Engage abdomen. Lengthen tailbone, tucking it toward the floor.

-   Exhale and sweep arms back down along sides of the body.

Standing Half Forward Bend

-   Begin in Standing Forward Bend. Push hands into the floor or against shins or knees. Inhale and straighten arms, lifting the torso away from the thighs.

-   Look forward slightly. Hold the arched-back position for one or two breaths. Exhale and release to Standing Forward Bend.

<u>Downward Facing Dog</u>

- Begin on hands and knees. Fingers spread wide on the floor or yoga mat. Fingers face forward or slightly turned out. Turn toes under.

- Lift knees away from the floor with an exhale. If hamstrings are tight, knees can stay bent and heels can be lifted. Lengthen tailbone toward feet slightly. Energetically draw legs in toward one another.

- Heels move toward the floor. Straighten through the legs as thighs push back. Upper thighs rotate inward.

- It is essential in Downward Facing Dog to have strong hands. Press the base of the index fingers into the floor. Lift inner arms. Shoulder blades draw together on the back. Head is neutral.

Three Legged Downward Facing Dog

-   From Downward Facing Dog

-   Bring feet together at the back of the mat. Keep arms and legs straight, inhale and lift one leg up. Flex lifted leg and reach through the heel toward the back of the room.

-   Internally rotate lifted leg to even out hips.

-   Keep the standing leg strong and keep shoulders squared to the front of the mat.

-   Keep head relaxed and in line with arms.

-   Hold for 5-10 breaths.

-   When ready, release lifted leg to the floor. Repeat with the other side.

<u>Triangle</u>

- From Mountain Pose, exhale and move feet about 4 feet apart. With hands on hips, turn your left foot in slightly to the right and right foot out to the right about 90 degrees. Firm up the muscles in legs.

- Raise arms to be parallel to the floor.

- Exhale. Extend torso forward, over the right leg, bending from the hip joint. Reach forward over your right leg, keeping the hips where they are. Left heel presses into the floor. Rotate the torso toward the left. Lengthen the tailbone toward the back heel.

- Right-hand rests on shin or a block outside right foot. Bring left arm up, reaching it toward the ceiling. Keep the lifted arm in line with the shoulders. The head can be turned up, eyes gazing toward the ceiling, or in a neutral position.

- Inhale to rise, pressing into the heel of the back foot. Reach through the lifted arm to fully rise. Switch feet and repeat on the other side.

<u>Low Lunge</u>

-   From Downward Facing Dog, lift right foot and bring it
    forward to hands. The knee should be over the heel.
    Lower left knee to the ground, turning the top of the
    foot to the floor.

-   Lift torso upright. Sweep arms up overhead. Draw
    tailbone down and draw the belly in. Draw shoulders
    down the back.

-   Gaze is upward. Reach fingers toward the ceiling.
    Hold for several breaths, exhale and return hands to
    the floor. Turn the toes under, lift the back knee and
    step into Downward Facing Dog. Repeat on the other
    side.

Low Lunge Twist

17

-   From Low Lunge, bring hands together and down in front of the heart.

-   Twist to the right, pressing the left elbow into the right thigh.

-   Press hands together, pointing the right elbow toward the ceiling.

-   Stay here for 3 - 5 breaths. To release, lift the torso until it is upright. Place hands on the ground, framing the front foot. Return to Downward Facing Dog.

<u>Standing Crescent</u>

- Beginning in Mountain Pose, join hands together, up overhead. Interlace the fingers and point through the index fingers. Press feet into the floor while reaching up through the hands.

- Relax shoulders down back as you reach up and out of the arms.

- Exhale and lean to the right. Keep feet evenly grounded and left hip pressing down toward the mat. Keep the leg muscles engaged.

- Remain here for at least 3 – 5 breaths.

- To release, inhale back to center.

- Repeat on the other side.

Tree Pose

- From Mountain Pose, shift weight onto the left foot. Bend right knee and turn the knee to face the right side of the room. Lift the heel and rest it on the ankle of the left leg. Stay here or, bend the right knee and reach down with the right hand to grasp the right ankle.

- Guide right foot up and place the bottom of the foot against the inner left thigh. Do not rest the foot on the knee joint. Toes point toward the floor.

- Hands rest on hips as the lifted foot presses into the standing leg.

- Hands come together in front of heart. Hands can press up overhead.

- Find a fixed point to gaze at. Stay here for 5 to 8 breaths.

- Return to Mountain Pose and repeat on the other side.

<u>High Lunge</u>

- Starting in Forward Fold step left foot back toward the back of the mat. Raise heel, keeping the ball of the foot on the floor. Right knee is at a 90-degree angle, the knee directly above the foot.

- Frame front foot with hands, laying torso on the front thigh. Come to a rise, tucking tailbone down and lift. Hands stay on bent knee or on the hips.

- Keep the back leg straight and sink into the front leg, stretching the groin and front hip.

- Exhale. Step right foot back to meet the left. Repeat for the other side.

<u>Warrior I</u>

- From Mountain Pose, exhale and step feet about 4 feet apart. With hands on your hips, turn your back foot in about 45 degrees or slightly more. Lining up the right and left heel, point the right foot forward, toes facing the front of the mat.

- Rotate torso to the right, trying to square hips to the front of the mat. Lengthen tailbone toward the floor.

- Bend front knee while keeping back heel down, toward the floor. Aim to bring right knee over your right ankle, the leg perpendicular to the floor.

- Inhale. Raise arms up, overhead, parallel to one another. Reach through the fingers without unplugging shoulder blades from the back.

- Continue to reach through the arms and draw the ribcage up and in, away from the pelvis. Lift the arch of the back foot remembering to keep the hips squared to the front of the mat.

- Either look straight ahead or tilt neck back, looking up at thumbs.

- Remain here for at least 5 breaths. To release, inhale and straighten the front knee and bring the back leg to meet the front. Return to Mountain Pose and repeat on the other side.

Warrior II

- Beginning in Mountain Pose. Exhale and step feet about 4 feet apart. With hands on hips, turn right foot so that the toes are facing the front of the mat. Turn the left foot toward the side of the room so that it is 90 degrees or parallel with the back of the mat. Engage the muscles in legs and turn left thigh outward, lining the left kneecap with the center of the left ankle.

- Bend left knee over the right ankle. Make sure that the shin and the thigh are at a 90-degree angle. If a 90-degree angle is not possible, bend as much as possible into the front leg. Keep the right knee stacking over the right ankle. Press the heel of the left foot into the floor.

- Raise arms so that they are parallel to the floor. Engage shoulders onto back while stretching arms away outward. Reach out in front and behind. Keep torso centered on hips.

- Press the tailbone down to prevent the low back from over-arching. Turn the head to the left and look out over the fingers.

- Stay for 30 seconds to 1 minute. Inhale to come up. Switch feet and repeat on the other side.

<u>Extended Side Angle</u>

-   Start standing in Mountain Pose. Step feet apart about 4 feet. With hands on hips, turn right foot so that the toes are facing the front of the mat. Turn the left foot toward the side of the room so that it is 90 degrees or parallel with the back of the mat. Engage the muscles in legs. Turn left thigh outward, lining the left kneecap with the center of the left ankle.

-   Keep the left hip rolling slightly forward so that hip points are facing down, but rotate torso so that it is facing back to the left.

-   Press the back heel into the floor and bend front knee over the ankle. Make the bend deep enough so that it is perpendicular to the floor.

-   Inhale and lift torso. Bring the right forearm onto the front thigh. Rest the arm here and extend left arm toward the front of the room, palm facing down.

-   Turn head to face the top arm and gaze at the palm.

-   Stretch from left heel through to the left fingertips.

-   Shoulders move away from ears. Stay long in the torso. Release right shoulder away from the ear.

-   Draw tailbone in and rotate torso more toward the ceiling.

-   Remain here for five breaths. Inhale to come up. Switch feet and repeat on the other side.

Chair Pose

-   Begin in Mountain Pose. Lift arms overhead on an inhale.

-   Exhale, bend knees and draw arms down, straight as they brush the floor. Thighs will be near parallel to the floor, and the knees will be closer to the front of the mat than the toes.

-   Lift the arms overhead or perpendicular to the floor while torso moves upright. The torso will not lift fully but should be at about a right angle with the thighs.

-   Slightly tuck the tailbone and put weight more on the heels of your feet.

-   Remain here for at least 3 to 5 breaths.

-   Inhale and straighten legs, folding forward to come out of this pose. Slowly lift the torso until fully upright and in Mountain Pose.

<u>Plank</u>

- From Downward Facing Dog, inhale and come forward until shoulders are over wrists and torso is parallel to the floor.

- Engage hands and energetically draw arms in toward one another. Spread shoulder blades away from the spine.

- Lengthen the tailbone toward the floor. Thighs press upward. Look straight down at the floor, just forward of fingertips. Engage abdomen.

- This pose can build a lot of strength. Try holding for increasing increments of time. If modifications are necessary, lower knees to the ground.

<u>Legs up the wall</u>

- Start by coming to a wall. Sit sideways at the wall with one hip touching. Bend knees so feet sit on the floor.

- Pivot body so that the buttocks are toward the wall and legs begin to go up the wall. As legs straighten and go up the wall, lay on the floor. If this is too much, move bottom slightly away from the wall.

- Lay torso comfortably on the floor. Tuck chin slightly in, toward the chest to lengthen out the back of the spine. With arms straight along the sides of the body, reach fingers toward feet, to bring shoulders away from ears.

- Close or soften eyes and stay here as long as desired.

- To get out of this pose, let legs fall to one side as the body turns on its side. Drop legs to the ground and lift torso using arms to push up.

Backbends

<u>Cobra Pose</u>

- Lie on the stomach. Bend arms so that hands are on the floor directly under shoulder or in line with lower ribs.

- Stretch legs back, toes pressing into mat. Lift each leg to internally rotate the thighs and lower down again.

- Spread fingers on the mat and hug elbows in.

- Press feet and thighs into the floor and lift torso. Keep the pubic bone pressing firmly into the mat as well.

- Pushing back with hands will lift torso further. Maintain the connection between the lower body and the floor.

- Draw tailbone down and do not overly engage the buttocks. Draw the navel in. Gaze is forward.

- Stay here for 3 breaths. Release the pose into the floor, turning the head to one side.

<u>Bridge Pose</u>

- Lie on your back. Bend knees, feet hip distance on the floor.

- Exhale and lift hips by pressing into feet and backs of arms. Tuck tailbone down, firming but not over engaging the muscles of your buttocks.

- Keep thighs and feet parallel.

- Join hands on the floor and roll slightly to each side. Tuck shoulders under your body slightly. Firm shoulder blades onto the back.

- Keep gaze forward; chin tucked slightly. Do not turn head to either side. Lift the pelvis while tucking the tailbone.

- Stay here for at least 5 breaths. Release by exhaling and lowering hips to ground. This pose can be done in a supported way if a block or bolster is placed under the hips.

Twists

<u>Seated Twist</u>

- Sitting in a comfortable position on the floor, place right hand on the floor in front of you and left hand behind you. Pull into the right hand as you exhale and twist to the left.

- Continue to pull with the right hand and push with the left hand to bring you further into the twist. Gaze can be to the left side of the room or over the left shoulder.

- Stay here for at least 30 seconds, twisting more with each breath. Release hands and face the front of the mat once again. Repeat on the other side.

<u>Supine Side Twist</u>

- Lying on your back, bring knees to chest. Inhale.

- Exhale and allow knees to fall to the right side. Rest knees on or close to the ground.

- Extend arms out, perpendicularly on the floor beside you. Turn head to gaze over your left shoulder.

- Energetically push left hip toward the front of the mat, slightly arching the low back.

- Stay here for at least 30 seconds. Inhale, exhale and draw the knees back in toward the chest. Repeat on the other side.

Seated Poses

Cross Legged Forward Fold

- Sitting on a blanket or block, cross legs in front of you.

- Spread weight evenly, lengthening head, neck, and spine.

- Reach arms up overhead, exhale and bend forward at the hips. Rest arms and head on the mat. If this is not possible, rest your forehead on your hands, a pillow or a bolster.

- Hold for at least 1 minute.

- To exit the pose, walk hands back until upright.

- Cross legs in the opposite way and repeat the pose.

Boat Pose

32

-   Sit on the floor, legs extended. Place hands on the floor in line with hips, fingers pointing forward. Press hands on the floor. Keep back straight and lift legs. Sit on sitting bones.

-   Bend your lifted knees, keep thighs at a 45-degree angle with the floor. If knees can straighten, do so.

-   Raise arms, bringing them in line with legs, parallel to the floor. Plug shoulder blades on to back and reach through the arms. If this is too much, use hands to hold onto the backs of thighs, or keep hands on the floor.

-   Breathe easy and engage core slightly. Gaze at toes. Start slowly, holding for 3 breaths. Increase as ability increases

-   To release, drop the legs and sit upright.

<u>Seated Forward Fold</u>

- Sit down on the floor with legs out in front of you. If necessary, use a blanket to prop your hips up slightly. Activate legs and feet by pressing through heels. Manually separate your flesh by rocking onto each buttock one at a time and pulling the flesh away from you. Concentrate on pressing the pinky edge of your toes toward you to internally rotate your thighs.

- On the floor beside hips, press hands into the floor. Lift through the sternum.

- Inhale and lean forward, keeping the hands on the mat slightly behind you. Bend from the hips and be careful not to round the low back. If you can, grasp onto the sides of the feet to draw yourself forward even more. Otherwise, use a strap to pull yourself forward.

- Try to pull your belly button forward so that it is touching the thighs. Lift and lengthen the torso on the inhales and release more fully as you exhale. As you move further into this pose, remember to keep your legs firm and press the backs of your thighs into the floor.

<u>Happy Baby</u>

34

- Lie on your back. Bend knees into belly.

- Grip the outsides of the feet with the hands and open
  your knees to either side of the torso. Draw them in
  toward armpits.

- Keep ankles directly over knees and flex through the
  heels. Push feet into your hands and hands down on
  feet.

Seated Side Stretch

- Sit in a comfortable cross-legged position.

- Raise your arms overhead

- Lower left arm to the floor as you reach right arm to the left, creating length in the right side.

- Plug right hip into the floor, being careful not to come up on the right side.

- Keep head in a neutral position, looking down toward the floor, or up under the right arm.

- Stay here for at least 30 seconds. When you are ready to come up, lift left arm to meet the right. Bring torso upright.

- Repeat on the other side.

Cat Pose

36

-   Start in hands and knees. Set knees hip distance apart and wrists shoulder width. Keep head in a neutral position, looking at the floor.

-   Exhaling, round spine toward the ceiling while keeping shoulders and knees in the same position. Allow head to release toward the floor. Gaze is toward the navel.

-   This pose is almost always paired with Cow Pose to warm up the spine.

<u>Cow Pose</u>

37

- Come on all fours. Knees hip distance and wrist shoulder width apart. Inhale and lift sitting bones and chest toward the ceiling. Belly sinking toward the floor.

- Lift head and look forward.

- Exhale and return to Cat Pose. Repeat, alternating from Cow Pose to Cat Pose, several times following the breath.

<u>Bound Angle</u>

- With legs out in front of you, sit comfortably on the floor. You may need to sit on the edge of a folded blanket. Bend knees, pulling heels in, toward the pelvis. Drop knees to either side, pressing the soles of feet together.

- Draw heels in as close to pelvis as possible. Using the first and second fingers and thumb, grasp onto the big toes of each foot.

- Sit upright, lengthening down through the tailbone. Keep the shoulder blades on the back and draw the belly in. Broaden across the collarbones.

- Release your thighs toward the floor without forcing the knees down.

- Stay here for 5 breaths or more. When you are ready to exit, gently pull the knees together using both hands.

Reclined Bound Angle Pose

- Starting in Bound Angle Pose, lower the back onto the floor by leaning on your hands, elbows and eventually, back. Bring torso all the way down and support head on a blanket if needed.

- Using your hands, rotate the inner thighs externally and press the outer thighs away from the torso.

- Widen the knees away from hips and sink groin in toward pelvis.

- Extend arms out to the sides and rest here for at least 1 minute.

<u>Child's Pose</u>

-   Begin on hands and knees. Bring big toes to touch, keep knees separate. Knees wide enough to fit torso between them.

-   Hips press back and rest on heals.

-   Arms may rest, extended in front or along sides.

-   Tailbone tucks slightly.

<u>Corpse</u>

- Lie on your back and draw knees into the chest. Inhale and exhale to release fully onto the floor.

- Close eyes.

- Feet should be relaxed and flop out to each side. Extend through heels to lengthen the legs and release to relax.

- Arms should be alongside the torso. Extend through the fingertips to draw the shoulders away from the ears.

- Draw the chin slightly in toward the chest to lengthen out the back of the neck.

- Release all organs by softening the tongue, ears, forehead, nose, and eyebrows. Relax the eyes and allow the brain to sink back against the skull.

- Remain in Corpse for at least 5 minutes. To exit, roll gently to the right side into a fetal position. Stay here for a few breaths. Push your hand into the floor to lift you. Let your head be the last to rise.

THE JOURNEY BEGINS

Sequences

We've created several sequences to get you started on your yoga journey. Refer to the previous section for detailed descriptions of the poses in each sequence. Most of all – have fun and enjoy the relaxation, strength, and flexibility yoga brings.

Sequence for Energy

This sequence will get you energized and feeling ready to face your day. We begin with a series of poses called Sun Salutations. Sun Salutations are a combination of poses designed to build heat in your body while increasing strength and flexibility. They are used to warm you up.

<u>Sun Salutations</u>

- Start in Mountain Pose at the front of your mat.

- Mountain Pose

- Forward Fold

- Forward Fold half lift

- Forward Fold

- Downward Facing Dog

- Plank

- Cobra

- Downward Facing Dog

*Repeat the Sun Salutations 2 to 3 times before moving into the rest of the sequence below.

When you are finished with the Sun Salutations, stop in Downward Facing Dog for 5 breaths. Come forward to the front of your mat. Come to a seat and continue with the rest of the poses.

<u>(Sequence for Energy cont.)</u>

Hold each of the below poses for
3 to 5 long, even breaths.

- Squat

- Plank or Forearm Plank

- Triangle Pose ***Repeat on both sides**

- Low Lunge Variation - hands may be rested on knee
  or hips. ***Repeat on both sides**

- Downward facing dog leg lifts to open hips ***Repeat
  on both sides**

- Standing side bends - Stand with legs wider than hip
  distance to protect low back Bend to each side

- Standing forward fold with hands clasped to open
  shoulders

Return to a seat and treat yourself to a Corpse Pose
before getting on with your day!

Strength and Flexibility Sequence

This sequence is a good all-around sequence. It builds strength and increases flexibility.

Warm up:

- 2 Sun Salutations ***refer to page 43**

Standing:

- Mountain Pose

- Tree Pose

- High Lunge

- Warrior II

    *When you come to the end of this standing sequence, switch sides and repeat.

Core & Seated:

- Boat Pose

- Cross-legged forward fold

- Boat Pose

- Crossed legged forward fold

- Seated forward fold

- Legs up the wall

- Hamstring stretch ***Repeat on both sides**

- Happy baby

- Thread the Needle Pose ***Repeat on both sides**

- Bridge Pose

- Supine Side Twist ***Repeat on both sides**

- Corpse

<u>A Little Bit of Everything</u>

This sequence is good practice that covers all the bases. Begin at the front of your mat.

Warm up:

- Mountain Pose

- Mountain Pose with arms raised

- Standing Forward Bend

- Standing Half Forward Bend

- Standing Forward Bend

- Standing Half Forward Bend

***Repeat 3X**

Standing: * Hold each pose for 3 - 5 breaths.

- Standing backbend with hands on low back, fingers pointing down

- Standing fold, fingers interlaced behind

- Tree Pose ***Repeat balancing on other side**

- Mountain Pose

- Chair Pose

- Mountain Pose

<u>A Little Bit of Everything</u>

48

Seated:

- Seated Forward Fold

- Boat Pose

- Bound Angle Pose

- Staff Pose

- Forward Bend

- Bridge

- Supine Twist ***Repeat on both sides**

- Hug Knees to Chest

- Corpse

Restorative Sequence

This sequence is a great way to prepare you for a wonderful night of sleep or help you wind down. Holding poses for 3 to 5 minutes at least.

- Seated Forward Fold
- Bridge Pose
- Legs up the Wall Pose
- Supine Bound Angle Pose
- Seated Spinal Twist ***Repeat on both sides**
- Supine Spinal Twist ***Repeat on both sides**
- Corpse Pose

Restorative Sequence

CONCLUSION

We hope you've enjoyed this introduction to yoga. Beginning a yoga practice can be challenging. Being gentle with yourself as a beginner and staying dedicated to the practice is no small feat. Remember, the more you practice, the better you'll get. As poses become easier, take yourself to the next level.

Finding yoga and creating a practice can be a life-changing experience, we are grateful to have been a part of your practice.

Namaste.

SAMPLE YOGA PLAN

The following is a 4 week sample yoga plan that you can use to begin to incorporate yoga into your life immediately. Feel free to adjust the days as you see fit. Remember, to listen to your body. This 4 week program provides a rest day every other day, however, if your body tells you that you need additional rest days, take them. Another alternative would be, instead of taking a second rest day, compromise and replace the normal sequence for that day with a relaxing series of Sun Salutations. This will give you the energy balancing that you're looking for without the intensity of a full sequence. Remember to listen to your body and enjoy the journey!

<u>Week 1</u>

<u>Monday</u>:
Sequence for Energy

<u>Tuesday</u>:
REST DAY

<u>Wednesday</u>:
Strength and Flexibility Sequence

<u>Thursday</u>:
REST DAY

<u>Friday</u>:
A Little Bit of Everything

<u>Saturday</u>:
REST DAY

<u>Sunday</u>:
Restorative Sequence

<u>Week 2</u>

<u>Monday</u>:
REST DAY

<u>Tuesday</u>:
Sequence for Energy

<u>Wednesday</u>:
REST DAY

<u>Thursday</u>:
Strength and Flexibility Sequence

<u>Friday</u>:
REST DAY

<u>Saturday</u>:
A Little Bit of Everything

<u>Sunday</u>:
REST DAY

<u>Week 3</u>

<u>Monday</u>:
Restorative Sequence

<u>Tuesday</u>:
REST DAY

<u>Wednesday</u>:
Sequence for Energy

<u>Thursday</u>:
REST DAY

<u>Friday</u>:
Strength and Flexibility Sequence

<u>Saturday</u>:
REST DAY

<u>Sunday</u>:
A Little Bit of Everything

Week 4

Monday:
REST DAY

Tuesday:
Sequence for Energy

Wednesday:
REST DAY

Thursday:
Strength and Flexibility Sequence

Friday:
REST DAY

Saturday:
A Little Bit of Everything

Sunday:
REST DAY or

Restorative Sequence

OWN YOUR JOURNEY

Now you've seen a sample 4 week yoga routine. Perhaps you feel it is time to take charge of your journey yourself. In the pages that follow, we've provided you space to mix and match poses that you've learned to create your own sequences. If you don't feel ready for this right now, that's fine. Those pages will still be there when you and your body are ready to shake things up. Yoga is an individual journey and is as much mental and spiritual as it is physical. So take your time and remember to breath.

Sequence Name: ________________________________

Pose 1: ________________________________

Pose 2: ________________________________

Pose 3: ________________________________

Pose 4: ________________________________

Pose 5: ________________________________

Pose 6: ________________________________

Pose 7: ________________________________

Pose 8: ________________________________

Pose 9: ________________________________

Pose 10: ________________________________

Sequence Name: ____

Pose 1: ____

Pose 2: ____

Pose 3: ____

Pose 4: ____

Pose 5: ____

Pose 6: ____

Pose 7: ____

Pose 8: ____

Pose 9: ____

Pose 10: ____

Sequence Name: ____

Pose 1: ____

Pose 2: ____

Pose 3: ____

Pose 4: ____

Pose 5: ____

Pose 6: ____

Pose 7: ____

Pose 8: ____

Pose 9: ____

Pose 10: ____

Sequence Name: _______________________________

Pose 1: _______________________________________

Pose 2: _______________________________________

Pose 3: _______________________________________

Pose 4: _______________________________________

Pose 5: _______________________________________

Pose 6: _______________________________________

Pose 7: _______________________________________

Pose 8: _______________________________________

Pose 9: _______________________________________

Pose 10: ______________________________________

9 781981 260102